How to Make a Woman Orgasm

15+ Secrets to Making any Lady has Multiple Orgasm Every Time plus Advice from Sex Therapists

Cheryl Bach

How to Make a Woman Orgasm

Cheryl Bach

Table of Contents

Chapter 1

Introduction

Sex is a healthy and essential part of life, but it can be challenging to ensure mutual satisfaction. This book is meant to help you unlock the secrets to making any lady orgasm every time. Female orgasm is a complex phenomenon, and nothing beats the satisfaction that comes from being able to provide intense sexual pleasure to your partner. Unfortunately, not everyone is an expert on how to achieve this elusive goal. This is why a comprehensive guide that provides practical tips aimed at helping people learn how to satisfy their partners sexually is essential.

The female orgasm is particularly tricky to achieve and is often looked over as less important than the male orgasm. However, it is crucial for women's overall sexual health, mental and emotional well-being, and in enhancing intimacy with one's partner. This book tackles each part specifically by providing essential insights into every aspect involved in achieving this achievement. We understand that the process could be a little intimidating and overwhelming for some, but this book is here to guide you with practical steps.

This guide provides a comprehensive overview of the female anatomy and detailed instructions on how to stimulate different parts of the body for maximum pleasure. We'll delve into various foreplay techniques, sex positions that work best for female orgasm, and tips for increasing sensitivity. The experts will provide counsel and guidance on common myths around female orgasm, debunking those myths that stand in the way of success.

Moreover, this guide doesn't just focus on physical stimulation but also dives into the importance of communication between partners and understanding each other's needs. This will create a safe environment for both partners to express their unique desires.

In the following chapters, we'll give you access to more than 15 secrets that have been proven to work consistently. These perspectives offer unique ideas and tips that are often overlooked but could work wonders in achieving an orgasmic experience. Along with these secrets, we'll also provide professional guidance, advice, and insights from sex therapist experts who have spent their careers helping couples achieve sexual fulfillment.

This book aims to empower both men and women in unlocking the secrets to achieving a fulfilling sexual connection. It is essential to note that there is no one size fits all approach to female orgasm, and every woman's journey is unique. Therefore, our guide offers various techniques and insights that aim to cater to different individuals' preferences and desires.

In conclusion, this guide is meant to be a practical, accessible, and comprehensive roadmap to help individuals seeking to enhance intimacy with their partners and improve their sexual relationships. We hope that you'll find the information contained herein invaluable tools on your journey towards realizing mutual satisfaction and creating an enjoyable sexual experience. So dive in and let's explore the world of female orgasm together, unlocking 15+ secrets and receiving expert advice from sex therapists that will make the process easier and more fulfilling.

Remember, the journey towards achieving a fulfilling sexual relationship is a continuous one. It requires time, patience, and an open mind, and this guide is here to provide you with the resources to keep moving forward. We hope that this book offers you a path towards greater intimacy and pleasure in your sexual lives.

Chapter 2

Understanding Female Anatomy

To truly support a woman in achieving an orgasmic experience, it's essential to understand the female anatomy. Women's sexual organs include the clitoris, G-spot, and A-spot. All of these areas play a significant role in achieving orgasm by receiving stimulation.

A Detailed Explanation of Female Anatomy

The Clitoral Complex:

Starting with the clitoral complex, the clitoris is a highly sensitive organ located above the vaginal opening, and its sole function is sexual pleasure. The tip of the clitoris, also known as the glans, contains about 8,000 nerve endings that receive stimulation to produce pleasurable sensations. The clitoris also contains two legs that run alongside each side of the vulva, forming a wishbone-like structure attached to the pelvic bone. When these legs are aroused, they engorge with blood and become more sensitive to touch.

The G-Spot:

Moving onto the G-spot, it is a highly erogenous zone located about 2-3 inches inside the vagina on the front wall. It can feel a little wrinkled or bumpy to the touch and is responsible for producing intense and deep orgasms. Grasping the G-spot requires a unique and delicate approach since it's not always easy to locate. Using a "come-hither" motion with the fingers can work in stimulating it. It is important to note that the G-spot is not always present in every woman, and some women may not experience intense pleasure by G-spot stimulation.

The A-Spot:

The "Anterior Fornix," also known as the A-spot, is another vaginal area that can lead to intense enjoyment when stimulated. It is located deep within the vagina just before the cervix. Compared to the G-spot, the A-spot is less well known, but it is a highly sensitive area that produces deep and pleasurable sensations when stimulated.

It's crucial to remember that every woman is different, and what works for one person may not work for another. Therefore, it's essential to communicate with your partner and understand her unique preferences and what works for her. Some women find direct G-spot stimulation too intense, while others prefer it. Therefore, it's essential to experiment and try different techniques and methods to see what works best for your partner.

How to Locate and Stimulate Them during Sex

When it comes to stimulating these erogenous zones, many techniques can be used during sex, including manual stimulation, oral sex, and using sex toys. For clitoral stimulation, using fingers in circular or side-to-side motions, or using a vibrator can do the trick. During intercourse, C-shaped positions work incredibly well since they provide direct stimulation to the clitoris while allowing for thrusting. Positions like woman on top or cowgirl with a vibrator is also an excellent way to stimulate the clitoris during sex.

For G-spot stimulation, use your fingers to curve upwards and inwards, or try using a specially designed curved toy like a G-spot vibrator. It's important to incorporate plenty of lubrication during G-spot play since the area may not be very wet naturally.

The A-spot is less talked about when it comes to stimulating women's erogenous zones but can offer a different type of pleasure. It's best to approach the A-spot gently with firm pressure while using a lubricant. Since the A-spot is located deeper within the vaginal wall, it's an excellent idea to use a sex toy explicitly designed for A-spot stimulation.

In conclusion, understanding female anatomy plays a fundamental role in sexual pleasure and orgasm. The clitoral complex, G-spot, and A-spot can all be stimulated during sex, in different ways, to produce intense and satisfying orgasms. Each woman is unique and has individual preferences when it comes to stimulation.

Therefore, it's important to communicate with your partner to understand what she enjoys and what works best for her. Experimenting with different techniques, methods, and positions can help you find what works best for you and your partner, which can lead to a more fulfilling and satisfying sexual relationship. In the next chapter, we will explore the different techniques and tips available to make sure your partner achieves multiple orgasms every time you pursue sexual intimacy together.

How to Make a Woman Orgasm

Chapter 3

Communication

Communication is essential when it comes to achieving sexual pleasure and orgasm. As the saying goes, "communication is key," and it's no different in the bedroom. In order to have a fulfilling and satisfying sexual experience, it's important to communicate with your partner openly about your sexual desires and preferences.

Asking for What You Want

One of the keys to good communication in sex is being able to identify what you need to feel good. It could be a certain position, type of touching, or anything else. Asking for what you want doesn't have to feel awkward or uncomfortable. Being open about your desires is an important part of a healthy sexual relationship, and it can even be fun. Start by talking about what you like in a general sense, and then get more specific over time. You can use positive affirmations such as "I love it when you touch me there," or "It would turn me on so much if you did this." This type of communication can be arousing and lead to a more intimate experience.

Encouraging Open Communication in a Safe Space

Sexual communication is often considered a taboo topic in our culture, which makes it hard for people to discuss openly. However, creating a safe space where your partner feels comfortable expressing their desires allows for a deeper connection. Make sure to listen with an open mind and avoid judgment. Validate your partner's desires even if they're not aligned with yours. Setting the stage for honest conversations about preferences without fear of judgement will make the experience much more pleasurable.

Cheryl Bach

It's important to note that communication is not just verbal. Ensure that physical body language is used to communicate non-verbal cues as well. Being able to read your partner's body signals and respond to them is key to a successful sexual experience. For example, paying attention to moans, breathing patterns and hand movements can guide your actions to know when to speed up, slow down, or change positions. It allows for intuitive behavioural feedback loops that enhance nonverbal communication with your partner.

Sex Therapist's Advice

The ideal approach is to create a safe and open space for conversations and encourage each other to express their thoughts and feelings about what they like and dislike during sex. This communication encourages people to learn and listen to their partners changing desires, make adjustments, and find new ways to enhance pleasure and orgasm.

In conclusion, communication is fundamental to sexual satisfaction and orgasm during sex. Encouraging open and honest conversation within a safe space enables both partners to identify what they want and need to experience pleasure, explore their desires and experiment in new ways. It can be challenging to have these conversations, but with patience, positivity, and validation, you can master it.

Remember, sex is about intimacy and connection, whether physical or emotional, and communication fosters this dynamic. Take time to learn how your partner communicates and encourage a healthy dialogue to achieve the ultimate goal of sexual satisfaction. In the next chapter, we will dive deeper into different techniques and strategies to enhance sexual pleasure, such as foreplay and arousal techniques.

Chapter 4

Foreplay

Foreplay is key to achieving stronger and longer-lasting orgasms. Taking time to engage in foreplay activates the body's pleasure centers and prepares it for arousal, allowing for a more satisfying sexual experience. Here we will explore why foreplay is important, and how to engage in it effectively.

Why Foreplay is Important

Foreplay is essential in preparing the mind and body for sexual intimacy. It signals to the brain that something pleasurable is about to occur and begins to increase blood flow to the erogenous zones of the body. These erogenous zones include but are not limited to: the neck, ears, breasts, nipples, clitoris, and vagina. Engaging in foreplay can help to reduce anxiety, increase pleasure and provide a deeper intimate connection with your partner.

Different Types of Foreplay

Kissing

Kissing is a simple yet effective way to start foreplay. Kissing releases oxytocin hormones that provide an emotional bond between partners. You can start with gentle pecks on the lips, gradually increasing pressure and duration until you feel comfortable exploring each other's mouths.

Touching

Sensual touch is also a great way to initiate foreplay. Begin by running your fingers gently over your partner's body, focusing on the erogenous zones. Touching helps to stimulate nerves and awaken sexual arousal in the body. Ensure that you explore each other's body slowly and tease.

Oral Sex

Oral sex is a great way of giving pleasure to your partner without penetrative sex. Oral sex should be done with enthusiasm and communication. Begin slowly and gently by kissing and teasing the erogenous zones around the genitals, then add pressure or indulge in different lingual techniques. Communication is key, and one should listen to their partner's verbal and non-verbal cues.

Dirty Talk

Dirty talk is a great way of expressing sexual desires and creating an intimate connection. You can start by whispering sensual words into your partner's ear during foreplay. It would help if you also asked what they like to hear or want to say. This communication will help clarify boundaries and desires between the partners.

How to Engage in Foreplay without Feeling Rushed

Foreplay should never feel rushed as it's supposed to be a relaxed and enjoyable experience for both partners. Here are some tips on how to engage in foreplay without feeling rushed:

1. **Start slow**: Do not speed things up. Take your time exploring each other's body.

2. **Communication**: Ask what your partner likes and dislikes and respect their choices.

3. **Set the mood**: Create the perfect environment that will allow you and your partner to relax and focus. Dim the lights, add some music, and maybe even light some candles.

4. **Switch it up:** Don't be afraid to try new things and switch up your routine. Keep things exciting by changing positions, trying new techniques, or incorporating sex toys.

5. **Don't be goal-oriented**: Remember, the goal is not to reach orgasm quickly but to enjoy the entire experience fully. Take your time and enjoy the journey!

Advice from Sex Therapists

They recommend that couples explore each other's bodies and take time to communicate their needs and desires during foreplay. Good communication builds trust between partners, making the experience more enjoyable for both parties involved.

Overall, foreplay is a crucial component of sexual intimacy and pleasure. It helps to establish a deeper emotional connection between partners and prepares the body for more enjoyable and satisfying sex. Experimenting with different foreplay techniques can also help increase sexual satisfaction and intimacy. Remember never to rush through foreplay, prioritize communication, and enjoy the experience. By incorporating these practices into your sex life, you can achieve stronger orgasms and create a more fulfilling sexual relationship with your partner.

Chapter 5

Enhancing Sensitivity

Enhancing sensitivity in the genitals is a critical part of sexual pleasure and satisfaction. In this chapter, we will explore different techniques for enhancing genital sensitivity, including lubricants, sex toys, breathing exercises, and mindfulness techniques.

Techniques for Enhancing Sensitivity

Clitoral Stimulation

Clitoral stimulation can be achieved in many ways, including rubbing, kissing, or licking. A vibrating sex toy such as a clitoral vibrator can also be used to increase sensitivity and pleasure in the clitoris. Experimenting with different techniques and sex toys can help to find what works best for you regarding clitoral stimulation.

G-Spot Stimulation

G-spot stimulation exists at the front wall of the vagina and is usually two inches from the opening. When stimulated, it can lead to powerful orgasms.

Using a curved toy such as a G-spot vibrator or dildo can help to enhance the sensitivity and pleasure of the G-spot. It is essential to listen to your body and experiment with different techniques and toys to find what works best for you.

Nipple Stimulation

Nipple stimulation can also be incredibly pleasurable for many women. Rubbing, licking, and gently pinching the nipples are excellent ways to stimulate them. Nipple clamps or suction toys can also be used to increase sensitivity and pleasure in the nipples.

Edging

Edging is a technique that involves bringing yourself or your partner close to orgasm, then slowing down or stopping entirely before reaching climax. This process can help to build sexual tension and enhance sensitivity, leading to more intense orgasms when the orgasm is finally reached.

Using Lubricants and Sexual Toys

Using lubricants is vital in enhancing sensitivity during sex. Lubricants reduce friction and increase comfort, making sex more pleasurable. They can be used during penetrative sex or while masturbating. There are different types of lubricants, including water-based, silicone-based, and oil-based. It is essential to choose a lubricant that works best for you and your partner.

Sex toys can also help to enhance sensitivity and pleasure during sex. Vibrators, dildos, and butt plugs are excellent toys to explore with your partner. Experimenting with different toys can help you find what works best for you and your partner.

Breathing Exercises and Mindfulness Techniques

Breathing exercises and mindfulness techniques can also help to improve sexual response and enhance sensitivity. Deep breathing exercises can help calm the mind and reduce anxiety and stress, leading to better sexual experiences.

Mindfulness techniques such as focusing on physical sensations during sex can also help to increase sensitivity and pleasure. By focusing on the present moment and the physical sensations during sex, you can increase your awareness of your body and the pleasure you are experiencing. It can be helpful to focus on the rhythm of your breathing and the sensations in your body while engaging in sexual activities.

In conclusion, there are many techniques for enhancing sensitivity in the genitals. Experimenting with different techniques, lubricants, sex toys, and mindfulness techniques can help to improve sexual response and lead to more pleasurable experiences. It is essential to keep an open mind, communicate with your partner, and listen to your body when exploring these techniques. By incorporating these practices into your sex life, you can increase your pleasure and satisfaction, and enjoy deeper intimacy with your partner.

How to Make a Woman Orgasm

Chapter 6

Different Sex Positions

The ability to experience orgasm can be greatly influenced by the sexual position used during intercourse. In this chapter, we will discuss different sex positions that can help to enhance sexual pleasure and increase the frequency and intensity of female orgasms.

Overview of Different Sex Positions

Missionary Position

The Missionary position is a common and straightforward position where the woman lies on her back, and the man enters from above. This classic position allows for deep penetration while also providing easy access to the clitoris.

Cowgirl or Woman-on-Top Position

Cowgirl or Woman-on-top position is where the woman straddles the man while facing him. The woman has greater control of the speed of penetration and angles that can lead to better G-spot stimulation.

Doggy Style

Doggy style position is where the woman is on all fours, and the man enters from behind. This position can also lead to deeper penetration and G-spot stimulation. The man can adjust his angle of entry to hit different spots inside the vagina or use his hand to stimulate the clitoris.

Spooning Position

Spooning position is where both partners lay on their sides, facing the same direction, with the man positioned behind the woman. This position allows for ease of clitoral stimulation and G-spot access through an upward angle.

Reverse Cowgirl

Reverse Cowgirl is similar to cowgirl position but with the woman facing away from the man. This position allows for deep penetration with the man's angle positioned directly towards the G-spot area.

Detailed Explanation of How to Perform Each Position

Missionary Position

To perform this position, the woman lies on her back while the man enters from above by positioning himself on his knees. The man then places his hands on either side of the woman's shoulders and begins to thrust into her. The woman can wrap her legs around the man's waist to increase intimacy and allow for deeper penetration.

Cowgirl or Woman-on-Top Position

To perform this position, the woman straddles the man while facing him. The woman can either be on her knees or hovering over the man. The man can gently guide the woman's hips to achieve the desired angle of entry. The woman can also use her hips to control the speed and intensity of penetration.

Doggy Style

To perform this position, the woman gets on all fours, and the man enters from behind on his knees. The man can adjust the angle of penetration to stimulate different areas inside the vagina. The woman can arch and lower her back to change the angle of entry or use her arms to stimulate her clitoris.

Spooning Position

To perform this position, both partners lay on their sides facing the same direction. The man positions himself behind the woman with his legs bent and knees slightly pulled up towards his chest. The woman can then raise one of her legs to allow the man to enter. The man can then use his hand to stimulate the clitoris.

Reverse Cowgirl

To perform this position, the woman straddles the man while facing away from him. The woman can either be on her knees or hovering over the man. The man can gently guide the woman's hips to achieve the desired angle of entry. The woman can also lean back for further stimulation of the G-spot.

Tips for Adjusting Angles for Deeper Penetration or Clitoral Stimulation

- By changing the angle of entry and depth of penetration, the man can stimulate the different areas inside the vagina. Experiment with different angles to find what feels best.

- The woman can use her hips to tilt her pelvis towards the man's penis to achieve deeper penetration.

- The woman can also raise her legs, place a pillow under her hips, or use a sex wedge to adjust her angle and allow for better G-spot stimulation.

- Use a sex toy, such as a vibrator, to stimulate the clitoris during intercourse.

- Incorporate manual stimulation, such as using fingers or a sex toy, during intercourse to enhance sexual pleasure.

In conclusion, trying out different sex positions can be an exciting way to increase intimacy, explore new sensations, and enhance sexual pleasure. By finding a position that works best for both partners, you can increase the chances of female orgasm and maximize the experience for both partners.

Chapter 7

Edging and Teasing

Edging and teasing are two techniques used to build sexual tension and lead to more powerful orgasms. In this chapter, we will explore how these techniques work, along with how to incorporate them into your sexual routine.

Explanation of How Edging and Teasing Can Lead to More Powerful Orgasms

Edging involves building arousal to the point of almost orgasm and then pausing or stopping stimulation just before climax. This technique can allow for a more prolonged and intensely satisfying orgasm when it is finally reached. By delaying the orgasm, it can also help to increase the overall duration of sexual pleasure.

How to Make a Woman Orgasm

Teasing, on the other hand, involves playing with your partner's senses through touch or verbal communication, building anticipation, and desire. The longer you tease, the more worked up your partner becomes, leading to a stronger release.

When edging and teasing are combined, the result can be incredibly powerful. By teasing your partner with a combination of verbal and physical cues, you can build up their anticipation and arousal, allowing for one of the most intense orgasms they have ever experienced.

How to Incorporate These Techniques in Your Sexual Routine

Start Slowly: When experimenting with edging and teasing, it is crucial to take things slowly. Start by building arousal through kissing, touching and foreplay. Build anticipation with each touch, stroke, or whisper until your partner is begging for more.

Try Different Strokes: When you are ready to start edging your partner, try different strokes or ways to stimulate their erogenous zones. Try varying speed, pressure and location to keep things interesting and build arousal.

Take Breaks: When you feel your partner is close to orgasm, take breaks. Slow down the stimulation, pause for a moment or switch to a different type of stimulation. This will help to build anticipation and prolong the experience.

Communicate with your Partner: Communication is key when it comes to edging and teasing. Pay attention to your partner's reactions and ask them what they like and don't like. Let them know when you are about to pause or switch up the stimulation.

Mix it Up: Incorporate teasing into your sexual routine to build up anticipation and excitement. Use dirty talk, touch, and eye contact to heighten arousal and build anticipation.

Tips for Building Arousal and Anticipation in Your Partner

Start Early: Begin teasing your partner before you even enter the bedroom. Send flirty messages or whispers throughout the day to build anticipation and heighten arousal.

Use Multiple Senses: Engage your partner's senses by using a combination of touches, sounds, smells, and tastes to create a more immersive sexual experience. For instance, use scented candles or incense, play soft music, and offer your partner some wine or other drinks to relax their inhibitions.

Explore New Techniques: Don't be afraid to try new techniques in the bedroom, such as using feathers or ice cubes to stimulate your partner's skin. These sensations can be intense and heighten arousal.

Pay Attention to Nonverbal Cues: Watch your partner's body language and verbal cues to determine their level of arousal. If they seem tense or guarded, switch up your approach or tone to help them relax and become more receptive to stimulation.

Indulge in Fantasy: Role-plays and fantasies can be a powerful tool for building anticipation and arousal. Talk openly with your partner about what turns them on and incorporate their fantasies into your sexual routine.

Incorporating edging and teasing into your sexual routine allows for a heightened level of sexual tension and anticipation, leading to more intense and satisfying orgasms. Remember to take things slowly, communicate openly with your partner, mix up your techniques, and pay attention to nonverbal cues. By following these tips, you can take your sexual experiences to new heights and make your partner orgasm like never before.

Chapter 8

Multiple Orgasms

Multiple orgasms, the pinnacle of sexual pleasure, is a dream for most women. The ability to experience two or more intense orgasms in one session can take your pleasure to new heights. In this chapter, we will discuss some techniques and tips that can enhance pleasure and encourage multiple orgasms.

Exploring Multiple Orgasms

Before we dive into techniques for achieving multiple orgasms, it's important to recognize that every woman's body is unique and experiences pleasure differently. As such, the exploration and experimentation of what feels good must come first. Communication with your partner to understand what she finds pleasurable or what might be hindering her pleasure is key. Exploring together in a non-judgemental and supportive environment is what sets the groundwork for achieving multiple orgasms together.

Techniques for Achieving Multiple Orgasms

Building up the tension: One technique for achieving multiple orgasms is to build tension and then release it. This can be done by alternating between slow, stimulating touches and faster touches on the most sensitive spots. By edging, or slowly building towards orgasm but then stopping just as the orgasm is near, and taking a break to come back later to continue, you are gradually building and releasing the tension, making it easier to achieve multiple orgasms.

Use Vibrators: Vibrators can help women achieve intense pleasure quickly and easily, which can increase the likelihood of experiencing multiple orgasms. There are different types of vibrators that can stimulate different parts of the body depending on what feels good. Consulting with your partner before incorporating a vibrator is best, to ensure that she is comfortable with it.

G-Spot Stimulation: The G-spot is an erogenous area located inside the vagina, about two inches up on the front vaginal wall. Stimulating the G-spot can increase the intensity of the orgasm and help a woman achieve multiple orgasms. Using either fingers or a G-spot vibrator, gently stroke, press and explore the area to see what feels best for your partner.

Relaxation and Mental Stimulation: The brain plays a crucial role in achieving multiple orgasms. Creating a relaxing environment and incorporating mental stimulation, such as erotica or sex talk, can help a woman get into the mood and open herself to sexual pleasure. It's important to have open and honest communication with your partner about what relaxes and excites her.

Encouragement to Explore and Experiment

Exploration and experimentation are key to discovering what feels good for you and your partner during sex. It's important to encourage your partner to take the time and explore her own body, and help her feel comfortable to share with you what feels good and what doesn't.

Trying out different sexual positions and techniques can introduce new sensations and increase pleasure, potentially leading to more powerful orgasms and perhaps multiple ones. Having an open mindset towards trying new things, while still respecting each other's boundaries and ensuring that communication is ongoing will help make exploring, experimenting and the journey towards achieving those multiple orgasms exciting.

Ideas for Prolonging Pleasure and Extending Playtime

Foreplay: Engaging in extended foreplay can boost your partner's arousal and help her achieve multiple orgasms. By taking the time to focus on the senses through kissing, touching, and oral sex you are helping to heighten sensitivity and extending the pleasure.

Variations in Rhythm and Pressure: Experimenting with different rhythms, intensity, and pressure during sexual stimulation can create new sensations for your partner. Varying your approach, from soft and gentle touches to firm and fast stimulation, can keep things interesting and help prolong the experience.

Self-exploration as a Team: Engage your partner in self-exploration as you watch or touch each other. This can be a titillating experience for both of you and can help your partner become more in tune with her body.

Kegel Exercises: Encourage your partner to engage in kegel exercises to strengthen her pelvic floor muscles. Stronger muscles lead to more powerful orgasms, which can lead to multiples.

In conclusion, achieving multiple orgasms can be an incredible experience for any woman. Remember that every woman is unique and that exploration and experimentation are key. By taking the time to build up tension, incorporating vibrators, exploring the G-spot, engaging in relaxation and mental stimulation, and varying pressure and intensity, you can set the groundwork for multiple orgasms. Encourage your partner to explore and experiment, try out different positions, and engage in extended foreplay to prolong pleasure and extend playtime. Remember to always communicate and respect each other's boundaries while never forgetting the importance of having fun.

Chapter 9

Common Sexual Myths

Sexual myths have been perpetuated for centuries, and unfortunately, they often lead to misunderstandings and confusion when it comes to female orgasm. In this chapter, we will debunk some of the most common sexual myths related to female orgasm and provide you with evidence-based information about what actually works.

Myth #1

Women Should Orgasm from Penetration Alone:

The majority of women are unable to orgasm from penetration alone, with the clitoris being the most important erogenous zone needed to reach an orgasm. Although penetrative sex can feel good, it is not enough on its own to make a woman orgasm. Examining alternative methods such as manual stimulation to the clitoris, oral stimulation and incorporating sex toys like vibrators can increase a woman's chance of experiencing an orgasm during penetration.

Myth # 2

Women Can Orgasm Every Time They Have Sex:

This is simply not true. Orgasms require a combination of physical and psychological factors, and reaching climax is not always possible. While some women may be able to achieve multiple orgasms with the right combination of stimulation and relaxation, it is not a given that every woman will experience an orgasm every time she has sex. Many factors like stress levels, medication, or hormonal changes can affect a woman's ability to orgasm.

Cheryl Bach

Myth #3

Women Who Can't Orgasm are "Broken" or Abnormal:

This myth is damaging and entirely incorrect. There are many reasons why a woman might struggle with achieving orgasm, including psychological factors like anxiety or depression, physiological conditions such as vaginismus and medications that can impact libido. None of these factors make a woman "broken." It's important to understand your body and what works for you, as well as being open to exploring other approaches that might help you achieve orgasm.

Myth #4

Women Who Can't Orgasm Just Haven't Found the Right Partner:

Again, this is a harmful myth. While a positive sexual connection and communication with a partner can certainly enhance sexual experience, it doesn't guarantee an orgasm. Many women struggle with sexual dysfunction due to non-psychological factors like low testosterone levels after childbirth or hormonal imbalances. It's important to seek out qualified medical advice if you are struggling to reach orgasm, rather than falsely assuming the problem lies with your partner.

Myth #5

It Is Only Possible For Women to Experience One Type of Orgasm:

There are various types of orgasms; the vaginal orgasm, clitoral orgasm, G-spot orgasm, and blended orgasm. Every woman's body is different, and while some women may prefer one type of orgasm over the other, it is possible for a woman to experience multiple types of orgasms. Expanding your sexuality experiences with your partner will open up many doors in terms of exploring what works best for you, whether that is through clitoral stimulation or experimenting with G-spot massage.

Myth #6

Women Lose Sexual Desire as They Age:

While it is true that hormonal changes and medical issues can affect sexual desire as women age, there is no age limit as to when women can have satisfying sexual experiences or even attain the first of orgasms. Communication with a partner and encouraging sexual intimacy through touching, kissing, and through self-exploration can help enhance sexual desire and keep the fire burning well into old age.

In conclusion, it is essential to be cautious about the sexual myths that we hear or read in the media. Many of these myths can be harmful and perpetuate damaging stereotypes around female sexuality. By understanding what the real truth is when it comes to female orgasm, women can have more fulfilling sexual experiences while feeling empowered and in control of their own bodies. It's important to take the time to explore different approaches, communicate with a partner, and seek out professional advice if needed. With patience, persistence, and an open mind, women can achieve multiple orgasms and experience sexual pleasure that is not inhibited by outdated misconceptions.

Chapter 10

Sex Therapy Advice

Sex therapy can be an incredibly useful tool for both individuals and couples who are looking to improve their sexual experiences. One of the main areas of focus in sex therapy is often female orgasm. Many individuals, particularly women, struggle to reach orgasm and may experience a myriad of frustrations, anxieties, and insecurities because of this. Thankfully, trained sex therapists are equipped with a variety of tools and techniques to help people overcome these barriers and find greater pleasure and satisfaction in their sex lives.

Advice from Sex Therapists on How to Approach Female Orgasm

For those seeking to improve their own orgasms or help their partner find greater pleasure, it can be helpful to consult professional advice. Sex therapists can offer a wealth of guidance on how to approach the topic of female orgasm, including specific techniques and approaches that can be used to help individuals achieve more satisfying outcomes.

Here are just a few examples:

-Communication: Many couples struggle to talk openly and honestly about their sexual needs and desires. Sex therapists can help individuals learn effective communication strategies and feel empowered to express their wants in a way that is respectful and affirming.

-Exploration: Sometimes, the key to unlocking greater pleasure lies in simply trying new things. Sex therapists can provide guidance on how to explore different kinds of touch, positions, and sensations to find what works best for each individual.

-Relaxation techniques: Anxiety and stress can be major barriers to female orgasm. Sex therapists can teach individuals relaxation techniques, such as mindfulness or deep breathing, to help reduce stress and anxiety and create a more conducive environment for pleasure.

Encouragement to Seek Professional Help When Needed

While sex therapy can be incredibly helpful, it's also important to recognize that some issues may require more extensive or specialized treatment. For example, some individuals may struggle with lifelong struggles or medical conditions like vaginismus or anorgasmia that require additional care. In these cases, sex therapists can provide referrals to other healthcare professionals who can offer more targeted support.

It's important to remember that there is no shame in seeking out professional help. Everyone has different needs and may require different forms of intervention or guidance to achieve their desired outcomes. By working with a trained sex therapist, individuals can gain greater confidence, trust, and pleasure in their sexual experiences, ultimately leading to a happier, healthier, and more fulfilling life.

Ultimately, the goal of sex therapy when it comes to female orgasm is to help individuals and couples experience greater pleasure and intimacy. This means approaching the topic with empathy, curiosity, and a willingness to experiment and try new things.

One approach that sex therapists often recommend is to focus less on the end result of orgasm and more on the process of exploration and connection. By helping partners learn to communicate effectively, explore new sensations, and create a relaxed and mutually supportive environment, sex therapists can help individuals experience greater pleasure regardless of whether or not they reach orgasm.

Overall, whether you're seeking to improve your own orgasms or help your partner experience greater pleasure, there are a variety of tools and techniques that sex therapists can offer. By opening up communication, experimenting with new approaches, and seeking professional help when necessary, individuals can find greater confidence, satisfaction, and joy in their sexual experiences and ultimately strengthen their relationships. It's important to be open to exploring different approaches and seeking out professional guidance when needed, as this can help individuals overcome any barriers or challenges that may be preventing them from experiencing greater pleasure and connection.

In conclusion, sex therapy can be an incredibly valuable resource for anyone who is looking to improve their sexual experiences and overcome barriers to female orgasm. By seeking out professional guidance and being open to new approaches and techniques, individuals and couples can enjoy greater pleasure, intimacy, and satisfaction in their sex lives. Remember, there is no shame in seeking help, and with the right support, anyone can achieve greater pleasure and connection.

How to Make a Woman Orgasm

Chapter 11

Maintaining a Healthy Sexual Relationship

One of the most important keys to maintaining a healthy sexual relationship is ongoing communication. This means being open and honest with your partner about your needs, desires, and boundaries, as well as being receptive to your partner's feedback and concerns. Keeping the lines of communication open can help prevent misunderstandings, build trust, and create a more supportive and loving environment for both partners.

The Importance of Ongoing Sexual Communication

Communication is critical to any healthy relationship, and this holds particularly true for sexual relationships. When it comes to sexual communication, honesty and openness are key. Partners should feel free to discuss their sexual needs, desires, and boundaries in a way that is respectful and affirming.

In addition to verbal communication, nonverbal cues can also play an important role in sexual communication. Paying attention to your partner's body language and reactions during sex can help you better understand their needs and desires.

Tips for Maintaining a Healthy Sexual Relationship

Here are some tips on how to maintain a healthy sexual relationship:

Prioritize intimate time together: In the midst of busy schedules and daily stressors, it's important to prioritize time for intimacy with your partner. This can involve scheduling regular date nights or romantic weekends away, or simply carving out some quiet time together each day.

Focus on mutual pleasure: In a healthy sexual relationship, both partners should feel heard and valued. Focus on mutual pleasure by exploring each other's bodies and experimenting with different sensations and techniques.

Be open to trying new things: Sexual preferences and desires can change over time, so be open to trying new things with your partner. This can involve exploring new positions, incorporating sex toys or props, or experimenting with new types of stimulation or fantasies.

Keep things fresh and exciting: Variety can be key to maintaining a healthy sexual relationship. Mix things up by trying out new locations, incorporating role play, or introducing new ways to connect emotionally and physically.

Strategies for Dealing with Sexual Issues as They Arise

Even in healthy sexual relationships, issues can arise from time to time. Here are some strategies for addressing these issues in a constructive and supportive way:

Avoid blaming or shaming: When discussing sexual issues with your partner, it's important to avoid language that is accusatory or blaming. Instead, focus on using "I" statements and expressing your own feelings and needs.

Seek professional help if needed: If you are struggling with sexual issues that are impacting your relationship, it may be helpful to seek the guidance of a sex therapist or other professional. These experts can provide a safe, nonjudgmental space to explore your concerns and develop strategies for moving forward.

Keep an open mind: Remember that sexual desires and preferences can vary widely from person to person. Keeping an open mind and being willing to explore new approaches or techniques can help to unlock new levels of pleasure and intimacy in your relationship. By remaining open to new experiences and staying curious about your partner's needs and desires, you can cultivate a healthy and fulfilling sexual relationship that continues to grow and evolve over time.

Address issues as they emerge: Ignoring sexual issues will only make them worse. As a couple, it is important to identify and address any concerns or challenges as they arise. This may involve having difficult conversations or working through difficult emotions, but by dealing with these issues head-on, you can prevent them from becoming morc cntrenched or causing further damage to your relationship.

In conclusion, maintaining a healthy sexual relationship requires ongoing communication, a focus on mutual pleasure and exploration, and a willingness to address challenges as they arise. By prioritizing intimacy, staying open-minded, seeking professional help when needed, and addressing concerns as they emerge, you can create an environment of trust, respect, and love that supports a healthy and satisfying sexual relationship for both partners.

How to Make a Woman Orgasm

Remember to approach sexual communication with honesty and openness, and to focus on mutual pleasure and exploration in order to keep things fresh and exciting. By staying curious about each other's needs and desires, and by working together to navigate any challenges that may arise, you can build a vibrant and fulfilling sexual relationship that deepens your connection as a couple.

Chapter 12

Conclusion

In this book, we have explored a range of techniques and tips for achieving maximum sexual pleasure for women. We've learned that while every woman differs in what stimulates her sexually, there are certain universal techniques that can help to bring about a satisfying orgasm every time. Additionally, we have gained insights from sex therapists, who have provided helpful advice and guidance on fostering a healthy sexual relationship.

Recap of the 15+ Secrets to Making Any Lady Have Multiple Orgasms Every Time

Let's recap some of the key secrets we've discovered on how to make any lady have multiple orgasms every time:

How to Make a Woman Orgasm

1. Take time to explore her body and learn what she likes

2. Communicate openly about desires and preferences

3. Focus on foreplay and building excitement

4. Use your hands and mouth to stimulate the clitoris

5. Experiment with different positions and techniques

6. Use sex toys and props to enhance pleasure

7. Pay attention to your rhythm and pace, matching hers to build tension

8. Be attentive and responsive to her cues and feedback

9. Incorporate variety and novelty to keep things interesting

10. Create a relaxing, comfortable atmosphere

11. Practice deep breathing and relaxation techniques to reduce tension and anxiety

12. Use dirty talk and other forms of erotic communication

13. Take breaks and switch things up to prevent overstimulation

14. Consider trying tantric or other holistic approaches to sexual pleasure

15. Remember that emotional intimacy and trust are key to a fulfilling sexual relationship.

Encouragement to Explore and Experiment with Different Techniques

By exploring and experimenting with these techniques, couples can achieve maximum sexual pleasure and mutual satisfaction. However, it's important to remember that every woman is unique, and what works for one may not work for another. The key is to remain curious and attentive to your partner's needs and desires, and to keep an open mind and willing spirit to try new things.

Final Words on the Importance of Prioritizing a Fulfilling and Mutually Satisfying Sexual Relationship

As a last word, it is imperative that partners prioritize creating fulfilling, mutually satisfying sexual relationships. A relationship that prioritizes sexual intimacy and pleasure creates trust, builds emotional connection, and ultimately fosters overall satisfaction in the relationship. It is essential to prioritize sexual communication, emotional intimacy, and a willingness to explore and experiment with new techniques for maximum pleasure.

Remember, the journey to female orgasm and sexual satisfaction requires patience, attentiveness, and empathy from both partners. With dedication and openness, couples can create a sexual landscape that is tailor-made for their specific needs and desires, leading to not just physical but emotional liberation and satisfaction. Cheers to a fulfilling sex life!

Chapter 13

Bonus

To add to the secrets already shared in this book, this chapter provides additional techniques that could help women reach orgasm. We will also explore real-life examples of women who have achieved orgasm through different approaches and provide answers to frequently asked questions about female orgasm.

Enhancing Pleasure with New Techniques

Learning to enjoy intimacy is an essential part of achieving orgasm. Using new techniques can spice things up and intensify the pleasure.

Here are some strategies to enhance pleasure:

How to Make a Woman Orgasm

Change Positions Regularly - Switching up positions during sex can keep the excitement level high. Adding new positions can also be a great way to explore different sensations and erogenous zones.

Gentle Touching - Sensuous touching can play a significant part in intensifying the pleasure of intimacy. A slow build-up of gentle touching, kissing, or caressing with different parts of your body, like your hands, lips, or tongue, can heighten a woman's chances of orgasm.

Experimentation - Trying out unconventional positions or exploring other untouched erogenous zones like the nipples or ears can add new levels of pleasure to intimacy.

Real-Life Examples of Women Achieving Orgasm through Different Approaches

Every woman's anatomy and pleasure points are unique. Trying out different approaches and discovering what works best can lead to consistent and fulfilling orgasms.

Here are some examples of real-life situations where women reached orgasm.

Nipple Play - For some women, nipple stimulation can bring them to orgasm. Gentle kissing, licking, or caressing the nipples during sex, can intensify sensations, leading to a powerful climax.

Oral Stimulation - Oral sex is a fantastic way to explore and achieve intense pleasure. Many women find that extra stimulation around the clitoris during fellatio or cunnilingus leads to orgasm.

Anal Stimulation - Some women may find that anal stimulation can lead to a more intense and pleasurable climax.

Dual Stimulation - Simultaneously stimulating the G-spot and clitoris multiplies a woman's chance of achieving an orgasm. This can be accomplished through manual stimulation, penetrative sex or with the use of toys.

Mental Stimulation - For some women, mental stimulation is an essential aspect of female orgasm, setting the tone for sexual arousal. Using erotic literature, intimate conversations or role-plays can stimulate the mind and lead to an unforgettable experience.

Frequently Asked Questions about Female Orgasm Answered by Experts

Can all women achieve orgasm?

Not all women have orgasms. Some may require a more extended time, more intense stimulation or particular methods to get there. However, trying new methods and techniques could help many women experience an orgasm.

How long does it typically take for a woman to achieve an orgasm?

The duration of achieving an orgasm varies from one individual to another. Some women may reach orgasm quickly while some may take more time, depending on various factors such as age, physical and emotional state, and experience.

Can a woman achieve a climax through penetrative sex alone?

While some women can achieve an orgasm through penetrative sex, a majority of women need extra stimulation such as clitoral stimulation to reach orgasm.

What is the G-spot, and does it play a role in female orgasm?

The G-spot is an area inside the vagina located about two inches in on the front vaginal wall. While there is still much debate among experts, some women find that stimulating the G-spot can enhance their sexual pleasure and can sometimes lead to orgasm.

Can medication affect a woman's ability to orgasm?

Yes, certain medications, such as antidepressants or birth control pills, can affect a woman's ability to orgasm by reducing libido or changing hormonal balances. Talking to a healthcare provider and adjusting medication can help overcome this issue.

Adding variation and trying new methods to enhance pleasure during intimacy can play a significant part in achieving female orgasm. Putting more effort, communication, and experimentation into sexual experiences can have long-lasting positive outcomes in relationships.